KET

DIET

Ketogenic Diet: Healthy Ketogenic Diet Guide to Lose Weight, Reset Your Metabolism and Heal Your Body

The Ultimate Keto Food Guide for Beginner

@ Justin Miles

Published By Adam Gilbin

@ Justin Miles

Ketogenic Diet: Healthy Ketogenic Diet Guide to Lose Weight, Reset Your Metabolism and Heal Your Body

The Ultimate Keto Food Guide for Beginner

All Right RESERVED

ISBN 78-1-990053-74-0

TABLE OF CONTENTS

Crock Pot Keto English Muffin 1

Crock Pot Turkish Breakfast Eggs 3

Bacon-Mushroom Breakfast 5

Cheddar & Bacon Casserole 7

Onion Broccoli Cream Cheese Quiche 9

Scrambled Eggs With Smoked Salmon 11

Garlic-Parmesan Asparagus Crock Pot 13

Crock Pot Cream Cheese French Toast 15

Cheese Grits 17

Pineapple Cake With Pecans 19

Potato Casserole For Breakfast 21

Chorizo Breakfast Bake 23

Baked Eggs In Avocado 25

Lemon Poppy Ricotta Pancakes 27

Sweet Blueberry Coconut Porridge 29

Sesame Pork Lettuce Wraps 31

Spiced Pumpkin Soup 33

- Easy Beef Curry 35
- Garlic Parmesan Cheesy Spaghetti Squash 37
- Skillet Cilantro-Lime Chicken... 40
- Buffalo Chicken 43
- Blt Lettuce Wraps With Avocado 45
- Chipotle Avocado Mayonnaise... 47
- Egg Muffins... 49
- Prosciutto-Wrapped Avocado With Arugula And Goat Cheese 51
- Garlic Butter Steak Bites.. 53
- Pesto Chicken With Burst Cherry Tomatoes 55
- Chocolate Fat Bomb Smoothie.. 57
- Creamy Tuscan Garlic Chicken 58
- Breakfast In A Glass... 60
- Amazing Keto Smoothie 61
- Low Carb Lunch Caesar Salad.. 63
- Amazing Low Carb Chicken Salad.................................... 64
- Delicious Keto Steak Salad 66

- Low Carb Fennel And Chicken Salad Recipes 68
- Keto Green Beans Salad 70
- Spinach Artichoke- 72
- Blackened Salmon With Avocado Salsa 73
- Blt Salad... 75
- Crab-Stuffed Avocado 77
- Grilled Halloumi Cheese With Eggs 79
- Creamy Kale Salad 81
- More Keto Recipes 83
- Greek Style Lamb Chops... 84
- Bacon-Wrapped Roasted Asparagus.............................. 86
- Keto Reuben Skillet 87
- Cauli Mac And Cheese.. 89
- Cheese & Pumpkin Chicken Meatballs........................... 91
- Cheese, Ham And Egg Muffins 93
- Beef And Kale Pan 94
- Chili Egg Pickles 96
- Gingery Tuna Mousse... 98

Creamy Cheddar Deviled Eggs 100

Pan-Fried Vegetables With Avocado Dip 102

Lasagne 104

Italian Vegetable Pan 107

Kohlrabi Fries 109

Coconut Thai Curry 111

Savoy Cabbage Stew 113

Pizza With Fresh Vegetables 116

Vegan Keto Pizza 118

Cauliflower Pizza With Salami 121

Pizza With Cheese Base 124

Crunchy Salami Pizza 126

Pizza Margherita 129

Avocado Lime Salmon 131

Rosemary Roasted Chicken And Veggies 133

Cheesy Sausage And Mushroom Skillet 135

Lamb Chops With Rosemary And Garlic 137

Keto Low-Carb Cheesy Tacos Skillet 139

- Keto Veggie & Fruits Smoothie 141
- Keto Iced Caramel Macchiato 142
- Peanut Butter Granola 144
- Keto Salted Caramel Hot Chocolate 146
- Keto Brownie Bark... 148
- Keto Pork Loin Roast With Herb Seasoning 151
- Lamb Chops With Rosemary And Garlic....................... 153
- Keto Low-Carb Cheesy Tacos Skillet............................. 155
- Keto Veggie & Fruits Smoothie 157
- Keto Iced Caramel Macchiato 158
- Peanut Butter Granola 160
- Keto Creamy Sun-Dried Tomato Chicken Thighs.......... 162
- Keto Ground Beef Stroganoff....................................... 164
- Pork And Mushroom Bake 167
- Juicy Pork Medallions... 168
- Pulled Pork With Avocado.. 170
- Buffalo Shrimp Lettuce Wraps 171
- Keto Bacon Sushi.. 173

Keto Burger Fat Bombs 175

Keto Taco Cups 177

Shrimp Salad With Yogurt Dressing 180

Keto Kale & Sausage Soup 182

Crock Pot Keto English Muffin

Ingredients:

- 1 large egg
- 1 pinch sea salt
- 1teaspoons baking soda
- Salt to taste
- 3 tablespoons almond flour
- 1tablespoon coconut flour
- 1 tablespoon butter

Directions:

1. Take a medium-sized skillet, melt the butter. It usually takes 20-30 seconds.
2. Pour coconut and almond flour, egg, salt into the melted butter and stir everything well.
3. Remove skillet from the heat and add baking soda.

4. Coat the slow cooker with cooking spray. Pour the mixture.
5. Put on low for 2 hours. Check the readiness with a fork.
6. Remove the baked muffin from the slow cooker and eat with bacon slices, cheese, or other breakfast staples.

Crock Pot Turkish Breakfast Eggs

Ingredients:

- keto bread 1 slice
- eggs 4 pcs
- milk 2 tablespoon
- small bunch of parsley, chopped
- natural yogurt 4 tablespoon
- pepper to taste
- olive oil 1 tablespoon
- onions 2 pcs, chopped
- red bell pepper 1 pcs, sliced
- red chili 1 small
- cherry tomatoes 8 pcs

Directions:

1. Grease the slow cooker using oil.

2. Heat-up, the oil, add the onions, pepper, and chili in a large skillet, then stir.
3. Cook until the veggies begin to soften.
4. Transfer it in the Slow Cooker, then add the cherry tomatoes and bread, stir everything well.
5. Cook on low for 4 hours, season with fresh parsley and yogurt.

Bacon-Mushroom Breakfast

Ingredients:

- Bell pepper, chopped - ¾ Cup
- Kale leaves large, shredded – 8 Nos.
- Ghee – 1 Tablespoon.
- Parmesan cheese – 1 Cup
- Avocado and green leaves Optional
- Bacon large, sliced – 4 Ounces
- White mushrooms, chopped – 3 Ounces
- Eggs – 6 Nos.
- Shallots, chopped – 3 Tablespoons

Directions:

1. Clean the kale leaves, remove the hard stems, and chop into small pieces.
2. In a skillet, cook the bacon till it becomes crispy, and add mushrooms, red pepper, and shallot.

3. Add kale and cut down the flame, and let the kale become tender in the skillet.
4. Now take a medium bowl and beat all eggs, add pepper and salt.
5. In the crock pot, add ghee and let it become hot. Spread the ghee on all sides of the cooker.
6. Put the sautéed vegetable into the base of the cooker.
7. Spread the cheese over the vegetables.
8. Then, add the beaten eggs on top.
9. Just stir it gently.
10. Set the cooker on low heat and cook for about 6 hours.
11. Serve hot with sliced avocado and green leaves.

Cheddar & Bacon Casserole

Ingredients:

- 1 green onion, chopped
- 1/2 cup milk
- Cooking spray
- A pinch of salt and black pepper
- 5 ounces hash browns, shredded
- 2 bacon slices, cooked and chopped
- 2 ounces cheddar cheese, shredded
- 3 eggs, whisked

Directions:

1. Grease your slow cooker with cooking spray and add hash browns, bacon, and cheese.
2. In a bowl, mix eggs with green onion, milk, salt, and pepper, whisk well and add to the slow cooker.

3. Cover, cook on High for 3 hours, divide between plates and serve.
4. Enjoy!

Onion Broccoli Cream Cheese Quiche

Ingredients:

- 1/2Tsp onion powder
- 3 cups broccoli, cut into florets
- 1/2Tsp pepper
- 1/4Tsp salt
- eggs
- 2 cups cheese, shredded and divided
- oz. cream cheese

Directions:

1. Add broccoli into the boiling water and cook for 3 minutes. Drain well and set aside to cool.
2. Add eggs, cream cheese, onion powder, pepper, and salt in mixing bowl and beat until well combined.
3. Spray slow cooker from inside using cooking spray.

4. Add cooked broccoli into the slow cooker, then sprinkle half cup cheese.
5. Pour egg mixture over broccoli and cheese mixture.
6. Cover slow cooker and cook on high for 2 hours and 15 minutes.
7. Once it's done, then sprinkle remaining cheese and cover for 10 minutes or until cheese melted.
8. Serve warm and enjoy.

Scrambled Eggs with Smoked Salmon

Ingredients:

- almond flour 1/2 cup
- Salt and black pepper
- Butter, 2 tablespoons
- fresh chives to taste
- Smoked salmon 1/2 lb.
- Eggs 12 pcs fresh
- heavy cream 1 cup

Directions:

1. Cut the slices of salmon. Set aside for garnish. Cut the rest of the salmon into small pieces.
2. Take a medium bowl, whisk the eggs and cream together.
3. Add half of the chopped chives, season eggs with salt and pepper.
4. Add flour.

5. Dissolve the butter over medium heat, then pour into the mixture.
6. Grease the Slow Cooker with oil or cooking spray.
7. Add salmon pieces to the mixture, pour it into the Slow Cooker.
8. Set to cook on low within 2 hours.
9. Garnish the dish with remaining salmon, chives.
10. Serve warm and enjoy!

Garlic-Parmesan Asparagus Crock Pot

Ingredients:

- egg 1 pcs fresh
- garlic salt 1teaspoon
- fresh asparagus 12 ounces
- Parmesan cheese 1/4 cup
- Pepper to taste
- olive oil extra virgin 2 tablespoons
- minced garlic 2 teaspoons

Directions:
1. Peel the garlic and mince it. Wash the asparagus.
2. Shred the Parmesan cheese.
3. Take a medium-sized bowl combine oil, garlic, cracked egg, and salt together. Whisk everything well.
4. Cover the green beans and coat them well.

5. Spread the cooking spray over the Slow Cooker's bottom, put the coated asparagus, season with the shredded cheese. Toss.
6. Cook on high within 1 hour.
7. Once the time is over, you may also season with the rest of the cheese. Serve.

Crock Pot Cream Cheese French Toast

Ingredients:

- sweetener 1 tablespoon
- milk 1 cup
- butter 2 tablespoon
- Cheddar cheese 1 cup
- Maple syrup, to taste, for dressing
- cream cheese 1 8-oz package
- slivered almonds 1/2 cup
- keto bread 1 loaf
- eggs 4 pcs
- almond extract 1 teaspoon

Directions:

1. Mix cream cheese with almonds in a large bowl.
2. Slice the keto bread into 2-inch slices.

3. Try to make a 1/2-inch slit horizontal at the bottom of every piece to make a pocket.
4. Fill all the slices with cream mixture.
5. Set aside. In a little bowl, mix eggs, extract the sweetener in milk.
6. Coat the keto slices into the mix.
7. Grease with cooking spray the slow cooker over the bottom and sides, then put the coated keto slices on the slow cooker's base. Put on the top of each separate piece additional shredded cheese.
8. Cook on low for 2 hours. Serve hot.

Cheese Grits

Ingredients:

- 1cup Cheddar cheese shredded
- tbsp butter
- Black pepper optionally
- 1cup stone-ground grits
- 5-6 cups of water
- 2 tsp salt

Directions:

1. Preheat slow cooker, spray the dish with cooking spray, or cover with butter.
2. In a wide bowl, mix grits and water, add salt.
3. Cook on low temperatures for 5-7 hours; you can leave it overnight.
4. Remove the dish from the slow cooker, cover butter on top.

5. Stir with the whisk to an even consistency and fully melted butter.
6. To serve, sprinkle more cheese on top and black pepper to your taste.
7. Serve warm.

Pineapple Cake with Pecans

Ingredients:

- 1 can pineapple with juice crushed
- 1 tsp baking soda
- 1 tsp vanilla extract
- Salt
- 2 cups of sugar
- 2 cups plain flour
- 2 eggs
- tbsp vegetable oil

For icing:

- 3tbsp shredded coconut
- 1cup chopped pecans toasted
- 1 cup of sugar
- 1cup butter
- tbsp evaporated milk

Directions:

1. Preheat your slow cooker to 180-200 degrees. Take a medium bowl and combine all cake Ingredients:.
2. Mix the dough until evenly combined and then pour into slow cooker dish.
3. Bake for 3 hours on high; check if it is ready with a wooden toothpick.
4. When the cake is ready, make the icing: in a medium saucepan, combine sugar, evaporated milk, butter, and salt.
5. Bring to boil, and then simmer with a lower heat for 10 minutes.
6. Add the coconut to the icing.
7. Put the icing over the hot cake, then sprinkle with nuts.
8. To serve, let the cake cool, then cut it and serve with your favorite drinks.

Potato Casserole for Breakfast

Ingredients:

- 5-6 green onions
- 10 chicken eggs
- 1cup milk
- Salt
- Black pepper
- 4 big potatoes
- 5-6 sausages
- 1cup cheddar cheese shredded
- 1cup mozzarella cheese

Directions:

1. Preheat slow cooker; spray its dish with non-stick cooking spray.
2. Rub the potatoes into small pieces and put them into the dish.

3. Cover the potatoes with rubbed sausages. Add both mozzarella, cheddar cheeses, and green onions.
4. Continue the layers until all space in the dish is full.
5. Mix the wet Ingredients: milk, eggs in a medium bowl.
6. Pour it into the main dish, then put salt and pepper.

Chorizo breakfast bake

Ingredients:

1 tablespoon olive oil

1 cup diced red pepper

1 cup diced yellow onion

4 ounces chorizo sausage

2 large eggs o Salt and pepper

2 slices thick-cut bacon, cooked

Directions:

1. Preheat the oven to 350°F and lightly grease two ramekins.
2. Heat the oil in a skillet over medium-high heat.
3. Add the peppers and onions and cook for 4 to 5 minutes until browned.
4. Divide the vegetable mixture between the two ramekins.

5. Chop the chorizo and divide between the ramekins.
6. Crack an egg into each ramekin and season with salt and pepper to taste.
7. Bake for 10 to 12 minutes until the egg is set to the desired level.
8. Crumble the bacon over top and serve hot. Makes 2 servings.

Baked eggs in avocado

Ingredients:

1 medium avocado

2 tablespoons lime juice

2 large eggs

Salt and pepper

2 tablespoons shredded cheddar cheese

Directions:

1. Preheat the oven to 450°F and cut the avocado in half.
2. Scoop out some of the flesh from the middle of each avocado half.
3. Place the avocado halves upright in a baking dish and brush with lime juice.
4. Crack an egg into each and season with salt and pepper.
5. Bake for 10 minutes then sprinkle with cheese.

6. Let the eggs bake for another 2 to 3 minutes until the cheese is melted. Serve hot.

Lemon Poppy ricotta pancakes

Ingredients:

1 large lemon, juiced and zested

6 ounces whole milk ricotta

3 large eggs

10 to 12 drops liquid stevia

1/2 cup almond flour

1 scoop egg white protein powder

1 tablespoon poppy seeds

¾ teaspoons baking powder

1/2 cup powdered erythritol

1 tablespoon heavy cream

Directions:

1. Combine the ricotta, eggs, and liquid stevia in a food processor with half the lemon juice and

the lemon zest – blend well then pour into a bowl.
2. Whisk in the almond flour, protein powder, poppy seeds, baking powder, and a pinch of salt.
3. Heat a large nonstick pan over medium heat.
4. Spoon the batter into the pan, using about 1/2 cup per pancake.
5. Cook the pancakes until bubbles form in the surface of the batter then flip them.
6. Let the pancakes cook until the bottom is browned then remove to a plate.
7. Repeat with the remaining batter.
8. Whisk together the heavy cream, powdered erythritol, and reserved lemon juice and zest.
9. Serve the pancakes hot drizzled with the lemon glaze.

Sweet Blueberry coconut porridge

Ingredients:

- 1/2 cup ground flaxseed
- 1 teaspoon ground cinnamon
- 1/2 teaspoon ground nutmeg
- Pinch salt
- 60 grams fresh blueberries
- 1/2 cup shaved coconut
- 1 cup unsweetened almond milk
- 1/2 cup canned coconut milk
- 1/2 cup coconut flour

Directions:

1. Warm the almond milk and coconut milk in a saucepan over low heat.

2. Whisk in the coconut flour, flaxseed, cinnamon, nutmeg, and salt.
3. Turn up the heat and cook until the mixture bubbles.
4. Stir in the sweetener and vanilla extract then cook until thickened to the desired level.
5. Spoon into two bowls and top with blueberries and shaved coconut.

Sesame Pork Lettuce Wraps

Ingredients:

- 1 tablespoon olive oil
- 1/2 cup diced yellow onion
- 1/2 cup diced green pepper
- 2 tablespoons diced celery
- 6 ounces ground pork
- 1/2 teaspoon onion powder
- 1/2 teaspoon garlic powder
- 2 tablespoons soy sauce
- 1 teaspoon sesame oil
- 4 leaves butter lettuce, separated
- 1 tablespoon toasted sesame seeds

Directions:

1. Heat the oil in a skillet over medium heat.
2. Add the onions, peppers, and celery and sauté for 5 minutes until tender.
3. Stir in the pork and cook until just browned.

4. Add the onion powder and garlic powder then stir in the soy sauce and sesame oil.
5. Season with salt and pepper to taste then remove from heat.
6. Place the lettuce leaves on a plate and spoon the pork mixture evenly into them.
7. Sprinkle with sesame seeds to serve.

Spiced pumpkin soup

Ingredients:

- 1/2 teaspoon ground nutmeg
- Salt and pepper to taste
- 1 cup pumpkin puree
- 1 cup chicken broth
- 3 slices thick-cut bacon
- 1/2 cup heavy cream
- 2 tablespoons unsalted butter
- 1 small yellow onion, chopped
- 2 cloves minced garlic
- 1 teaspoon minced ginger
- 1 teaspoon ground cinnamon

Directions:

1. Melt the butter in a large saucepan over medium heat.

2. Add the onions, garlic and ginger and cook for 3 to 4 minutes until the onions are translucent.
3. Stir in the spices and cook for 1 minute until fragrant. Season with salt and pepper.
4. Add the pumpkin puree and chicken broth then bring to a boil.
5. Reduce heat and simmer for 20 minutes then remove from heat.
6. Puree the soup using an immersion blender then return to heat and simmer for 20 minutes.
7. Cook the bacon in a skillet until crisp then remove to paper towels to drain.
8. Add the bacon fat to the soup along with the heavy cream.
9. Crumbled the bacon over top to serve.

Easy Beef Curry

Ingredients:

- 1cups canned coconut milk
- 1 pound beef chuck, chopped
- 1 cup fresh chopped cilantro
- 1 medium yellow onion, chopped
- 1 tablespoon minced garlic
- 1 tablespoon grated ginger
- 2 tablespoons curry powder
- 1 teaspoon salt

Directions:

1. Combine the onion, garlic and ginger in a food processor and blend into a paste.
2. Transfer the paste to a saucepan and cook for 3 minutes on medium heat.
3. Stir in the coconut milk then simmer gently for 10 minutes.

4. Add the chopped beef along with the curry powder and salt.
5. Stir well then simmer, covered, for 20 minutes.
6. Remove the lid and simmer for another 20 minutes until the beef is cooked through.
7. Adjust seasoning to taste and garnish with fresh chopped cilantro.

Garlic Parmesan Cheesy Spaghetti Squash

Ingredients:

- Low-moisture whole-milk shredded mozzarella cheese 3 ounces
- Parmesan cheese divided 2 ounces
- Fresh chopped parsley leaves 2 tbsp.
- Garlic powder 1tsp
- Cream cheese 2 ounces
- Spaghetti squash 2 medium
- Olive oil 1 tbsp.
- Kosher salt 1/4teaspoon
- Black pepper freshly ground 1/2tsp

Directions:

1. Place a rack in the center of the oven and heat to 400 ° F. Set up a parchment paper or aluminum foil rimmed baking sheet; set aside. In a large pan, put 2 ounces of cream cheese

and, at room temperature, let it rest until smooth while the oven heats up.
2. Lengthwise break in half.
3. Two spaghetti squash and pick the seeds out. Blend 1 tbsp.
4. of olive oil on the squash cut side and season with 1/4tsp kosher salt and 1/2tsp black pepper.
5. Arrange the cut-side squash into the baking dish. When poked with a fork, roast until the squash is tender and the skin is blistered and browned, around 40 min.
6. Shred 3 ounces of mozzarella cheese and grind 2 ounces of Parmesan cheese.
7. Cut, so you have two tbsp. of fresh parsley leaves and garnish.
8. Apply the mozzarella, Parmesan 1/4cup for topping, set aside the leftover 1/2cup, 2 tbsp.

9. of parsley, and garlic powder 1tsp to the cream cheese and mix with a rubber spatula to mix.
10. The baking sheet is withdrawn from the oven. Turn the squash over using a fork for shredding about half of the squash's interior, leaving unshredded squash only 1inch in the wrapper.
11. Pass the sliced squash to the combination of cream cheese, and swirl to combine.
12. Split the filling equally between the halves of squash, then scatter with the remaining quarter cup of Parmesan.
13. Bake for 8 - 10 minutes till the cheese is smelted.
14. Switch on the oven & broil until bubbly and browned another 2 or 3 mins.
15. Garnish more with parsley, then serve hot.

Skillet Cilantro-Lime Chicken

Ingredients:

- Garlic minced 2 cloves
- Medium limes 2 finely grated zest
- Lime juice freshly squeezed 1/2cup
- Freshly chopped cilantro leaves & tender stems 1/4 cup
- Optional for serving cooked rice
- Olive oil 1 tbsp.
- Chicken breasts 4 boneless skinless
- Kosher salt
- Ground freshly black pepper
- Unsalted butter 2 tbsp.

Directions:

1. Dry the chicken using paper towels.
2. Season properly with pepper and salt.

3. Steam 1 tbsp. of the oil over medium to high shimmering steam in a ten-inch or larger skillet.
4. If possible, working in batches, add the chicken and sear to the bottom for 5 to 7 minutes, until deeply browned.
5. Flip the meat, then sear for 5 to 7 mins before the other side is browned.
6. Place the chicken into a plate; put aside.
7. Reduce to medium heat.
8. Attach the garlic, butter, and lime zest, then cook for 1 minute, stirring frequently.
9. Stir in the juice of the lime.
10. Send the chicken back to the skillet and any leftover juices.
11. Cover, heat is reduced as required to maintain a moderate simmer and cook until the meat is cooked through and record 165ºF on thermometer instant-read, 2 to 3 min.

12. Stir some of the sauce and the cilantro and pour over the chicken.
13. When desired, eat with rice.

Buffalo Chicken

Ingredients:

- Ghee or unsalted butter 4 tbsp.
- Boneless chicken breasts 2 1pounds skinless
- Bottle hot sauce 1 12-ounce

Directions:

1. In a 6-quarter or Electric Pressure Cooker, a bigger Instant Pot put 2 1pounds of chicken breasts boneless, skinless into one layer.
2. Pour 1 12-ounce spicy chicken sauce bottle over it.
3. Cube 4 tbsp. of ghee or unsalted butter, then put the chicken on top.
4. Lock the cover in place and ensure that the valve is shut.
5. High pressure cooking to cook for about 15 minutes.

6. It's going to take 10 - 12 minutes to work up under pressure.
7. Once the time for cooking is finished, let the pressure drop for 5 min naturally.
8. Release the remaining pressure
9. Move the chicken right away to a clean cutting plate.
10. For slice the meat, using two forks, then move to a dish.
11. Whisk the sauce once mixed and emulsified in a pressure cooker.
12. Apply to chicken 1 cup sauce and flip to coat.
13. Apply more sauce if appropriate and set aside any leftover sauce to consume or store.

BLT Lettuce Wraps with Avocado

Ingredients:

- Squeezed freshly lemon juice 1 tbsp.
- Black pepper ground freshly 1/8 tsp
- Grape tomatoes half or pint cherry 1
- Diced avocado 1 med
- From 1 med head butter lettuce 8 leaves, like Bibb or Boston
- Bacon 6 slices
- Mayonnaise 2 tbsp.
- Fine chopped chives 1 tbsp.

Directions:

1. Set up a rack in the bottom third of the oven and to 400 ° F heat it.
2. Lined a baking sheet with aluminum foil or parchment paper.

3. Place the bacon in one layer onto the baking sheet. Bake 15 to 20 mins until crispy and rich golden-brown.
4. From the oven, Remove and allow cool. Alternatively, in a shallow pot, mix the mayonnaise, lemon juice, chives, and pepper; set aside.
5. Move the bacon to a cutting board until it's cold and chop it roughly.
6. Load a single leaf of lettuce with tomatoes, avocado, and bacon.
7. Drizzle with the dressing, then serve.

Chipotle Avocado Mayonnaise

Ingredients:

- Dijon mustard 1 tsp
- Lemon juice freshly squeezed 1 tsp
- Kosher salt 1tsp
- Olive oil 1/2cup
- Medium avocados 2 rip
- Chipotle chili canned finely chopped in adobo sauce 1 tsp

Directions:

1. In a mini food processor or blender, place the chipotle chili, avocados, adobo sauce, lemon juice, Dijon mustard, and kosher salt.
2. Process until smooth, for 30 - 1 minute. Scrape the bowl or pitcher side. Switch on the machine and drizzle gradually into the oil.

Blend, about 1 minute, until smooth & emulsified.

Egg Muffins

Ingredients:

- Large eggs 10
- Kosher salt 1 teaspoon
- Black pepper freshly ground 1/2tsp
- Olive oil or Cooking spray
- Sweet potato shredded 1 1cups
- Cheddar cheese shredded sharp 1 cup
- Strips bacon sugar-free, crumbled 6 cooked

Directions:

1. Arrange a middle-rack in -oven and to 400 ° F heat.
2. Coat a regular 12 well muffin tray generously with olive oil or cooking spray.
3. Divide the sliced sweet potato, bacon, and cheese equally throughout the wells of muffins.

4. In a large cup, put the eggs, half-&-a-half, pepper, and salt and whisk until the eggs are thoroughly integrated.
5. Pour in the wells of the muffins, filling 1to 1/4complete each.
6. Bake for 12 - 14 minutes until the muffins are set and brown slightly around the edges.
7. On a wire rack, place the pan and allow it to cool for 2 - 3 mins.
8. Run the butter knife to the release of the muffins around cups, each of them before extracting them.
9. Serve cold or warm, before cooling or freezing, absolutely on a wire rack.

Prosciutto-Wrapped Avocado with Arugula and Goat Cheese

Ingredients:

- Kosher salt 1/2tsp
- Prosciutto 8 thin slices
- Arugula 1 1cups
- Thinly sliced avocados ripe medium 2
- Goat cheese fresh 4 ounces
- Lemon juice freshly squeezed 2 tbsp.
- Black pepper freshly ground 1tsp

Directions:
1. In a shallow pot, mix the goat cheese, lemon juice, salt, and pepper until smooth.
2. Place pieces of the prosciutto.
3. Layer a single slice of prosciutto with 2 - 3 tsp of goat cheese mixture.

4. Split the arugula into the prosciutto, placing the greens on one end of each piece.
5. Cover each pile of greens similarly with 2–3 slices of avocado.
6. Operating with one prosciutto slice at a time, then wrapping up into a compact package beginning with the avocado from the end.

Garlic Butter Steak Bites

Ingredients:

- Thick-cut strip steaks New York 2 pounds
- Kosher salt 1teaspoon
- Unsalted butter 8 tablespoons
- Garlic 4 cloves
- Black pepper freshly ground 1teaspoon
- Parsley leaves chopped fresh 1/2cup

Directions:

1. Mince 4 cloves of garlic.
2. Place in a cup and apply 1tsp of black pepper freshly ground.
3. Cut until 1/2cup of fresh parsley leaves is available, then move to a small pot.
4. Cut 2 pounds of strip steak New York into 1-inch pieces, then apply 1tsp of kosher salt to season.

5. Melt 8 tbsp. 1 stick of unsalted butter over medium-high heat in a large skillet.
6. Attach the steak cubes, then sear until browned, tossing them halfway through, taking 6 - 8 mins.
7. Add the pepper and garlic, and simmer for another 1 minute.
8. Take off the heat and with the parsley garnish.

Pesto Chicken with Burst Cherry Tomatoes

Ingredients:

- Black pepper freshly ground 1/2tsp
- Chicken breasts boneless, skinless 4
- Basil pesto 1/2cup
- Grape tomatoes or pints cherry 2
- Olive oil 1 tbsp.
- Kosher salt 1tsp

Directions:

1. Place a rack in the center of the oven and to 400 ° F heat the oven.
2. Put the tomatoes on a baking sheet, which is rimmed.
3. Remove the grease, season with pepper and salt, and mix.
4. Spread out over a single sheet.

5. Pat, the chicken, completely dries it with paper towels. Season with pepper and salt. Put the chicken on the baking sheet in the middle.
6. Spread the pesto on each chicken breast about 1 tbsp.
7. each, spread on a thin layer, so each breast is covered evenly and fully.
8. Roast until caramelized the tomatoes have, and others have burst and cooked the chicken and registers 165 ° F, 25 - 30 mins, on a thermometer. Serve the drizzled chicken and tomatoes with pan juices.

Chocolate Fat Bomb Smoothie

Ingredients:

- Fruit sweetener 2 tbsp. 24g
- MCT oil powder 1 scoop 10g
- No-sugar-added Sun butter 1 tbsp. 16g
- Unsweetened cocoa powder 1 tbsp. 5g
- Salt 1/16 tsp
- Ice cubes 2
- Unsweetened coconut milk 1 cup 120ml
- Coconut cream 1/2 cup 60g

Directions:

1. Mix all Ingredients: and blend until well-blended

Creamy Tuscan Garlic Chicken

Ingredients:

- Garlic powder 0.67 tsp
- Italian seasoning 0.67 tsp
- Parmesan cheese 0.33 cup
- Spinach chopped 0.67 cup
- Sun-dried tomatoes 0.33 cup
- 1-pound boneless chicken
- Olive oil 1.33 tbsp.
- Heavy cream 0.67 cup
- Chicken broth 0.33 cup

Directions:

1. Put olive oil in a wide skillet & cook chicken on medium heat for 3-5 min on either side or until crispy on either side & cooked until the middle is no longer pink.

2. Place the chicken on the plate and put it aside.
3. Replace the whipping cream, chicken stock, garlic powder, parmesan cheese, and Italian seasoning. Whisk across moderate heat flame before thickening begins.
4. Connect the spinach & sun-dried tomatoes & enable them to cook before the spinach begins to wilt.
5. If needed, move chicken back to saucepan & serve over pasta.

Breakfast In A Glass

Ingredients:

- 1/2 cup cocoa nibs
- 1/2 cup cocoa powder
- 1/2 teaspoon turmeric
- 1 small avocado, pitted and peeled
- 1 cup favorite greens
- 10 ounces canned coconut milk
- 1 cup water
- 1 cup cherries, frozen

Directions:

1. In your blender, mix coconut milk with avocado, cocoa powder, cherries and turmeric and blend well.
2. Add water, greens and cocoa nibs, blend for 2 minutes more, pour into glasses and serve.
3. Enjoy!

Amazing keto Smoothie

Ingredients:

- 1 teaspoon whey protein
- 1 teaspoon green powder
- 1 tablespoon potato starch
- 1 tablespoon psyllium seeds
- 1 cup coconut milk
- 10 almonds
- 2 brazil nuts
- 2 cups spinach leaves

Directions:

1. 1.In your blender, mix spinach with brazil nuts, coconut milk and almonds and blend well.
2. 2.Add green powder, whey protein, potato starch and psyllium seeds and blend well again.

3. 3.Pour into a tall glass and consume for breakfast.
4. Enjoy!

Low carb Lunch Caesar Salad

Ingredients:

- 3 tablespoons creamy Caesar dressing
- 1 chicken breast, grilled and shredded
- 1 cup bacon, cooked and crumbled
- Salt and black pepper to the taste
- 1 avocado, pitted, peeled and sliced

Directions:

1. 1.Mix avocado with bacon and chicken breast in a salad bowl and stir.
2. 2.Then add Caesar dressing, toss to coat, salt and pepper, divide into 2 bowls and serve.
3. Enjoy!

Amazing low carb Chicken Salad

Ingredients:

- 1 tablespoons dill relish
- Salt and black pepper to the taste
- 5 ounces chicken breast, roasted and chopped
- 1/4 cup mayonnaise
- 1 teaspoon mustard
- A pinch of granulated garlic
- 1 celery rib, chopped
- 1 green onion, chopped
- 1 egg, hard-boiled, peeled and chopped
- 2 tablespoons parsley, chopped

Directions:

1. Mix parsley in your food processor with onion and celery and pulse well.
2. Place these to a bowl and leave aside for now.

3. Put chicken in food processor, add to the bowl with the veggies and blend well
4. Add eggs, salt and pepper and stir.
5. Also add mustard, dill relish, mayo and granulated garlic, toss to coat and serve right away.
6. Enjoy!

Delicious keto Steak Salad

Ingredients:

- 6 ounces sweet onion, chopped
- 3 ounces sun-dried tomatoes, chopped
- 1 yellow bell pepper, sliced
- 1 teaspoon Italian seasoning
- 1 teaspoon red pepper flakes
- 1 orange bell pepper, sliced
- 1 teaspoon onion powder
- 3 tablespoons avocado oil
- Salt and black pepper to the taste
- 1 and 1 pound steak, thinly sliced
- 2 garlic cloves, minced
- 1/2 cup balsamic vinegar
- 1 lettuce head, chopped
- 4 ounces mushrooms, sliced

- 1 avocado, pitted, peeled and sliced

Directions:

1. Mix steak pieces with some salt, balsamic vinegar and pepper, toss to coat and leave aside for now.
2. Heat up a pan with the avocado oil, add mushrooms, garlic, salt, pepper and onion, stir and cook for 20 minutes.
3. In a dish mix lettuce leaves with orange and yellow bell pepper, sun dried tomatoes and avocado and stirred.
4. Season steak pieces with pepper flakes, onion powder and Italian seasoning.
5. Place steak pieces in a boiling pan, then put in a preheated broiler and cook for 5 minutes.
6. Place steak pieces on plates, add salad on the side and top everything with mushroom and onion mix.
7. Enjoy!

Low carb Fennel and Chicken Salad recipes

Ingredients:

- 1/2 cup mayonnaise
- 2 tablespoons lemon juice
- 2 tablespoons fennel fronds, chopped
- A pinch of cayenne pepper
- Salt and black pepper to the taste
- 2 tablespoons walnut oil
- 1/2 cup walnuts, toasted and chopped
- 3 chicken breasts, boneless, skinless, cooked and chopped
- 1 and 1 cup fennel, chopped

Directions:

1. Mix fennel with chicken and walnuts in a bowl and stir.

2. Mix mayo with pepper, salt, fennel fronds, lemon juice, walnut oil, cayenne and garlic in a new bowl and stir well.
3. Put this over chicken and fennel mix, coat well and keep in the fridge.
4. Enjoy!

Keto Green Beans Salad

Ingredients:

- 2 pounds green beans
- 4 ounces goat cheese, crumbled
- 1 and 1 cups fennel, thinly sliced
- ¾ cup walnuts, toasted and chopped
- 1 and 1 tablespoons mustard
- Salt and black pepper to the taste
- 2 tablespoons white wine vinegar
- 1/4 cup extra virgin olive oil

Directions:

1. Pour water in a pot, add some salt and bring to a boil over medium high heat.
2. Add green beans, cook for 5 minutes and place them to a bowl filled with ice water.
3. Drain water from green beans well and put them in a salad bowl.

4. Add fennel, walnuts and goat cheese and toss.
5. Mix vinegar with mustard in a bowl then salt, pepper and oil and whisk well.
6. Put this over salad, toss and coat well and serve for lunch.

Spinach Artichoke-

Ingredients:

- 2 tsp. extra virgin olive oil
- Sea salt & pepper, to taste
- 1 1/2lbs. chicken breasts, boneless & skinless
- 1 tbsp. garlic & herb seasoning mix

Directions:

1. Heat a grill pan or your grill.
2. Coat the chicken breasts in a little bit of olive oil and then sprinkle the seasoning mixture onto them, rubbing it in.
3. Cook the chicken for about eight minutes per side and make sure the chicken has reached an internal temperature of 165°.
4. Serve hot with your favorite sides!

Blackened Salmon with Avocado Salsa

Ingredients:

- 1 c. cucumber, diced
- 1/2c. red onion, diced
- 1 tbsp. parsley, chopped
- 1 tbsp. lime juice
- Sea salt & pepper, to taste
- 1 tbsp. extra virgin olive oil
- 4 filets of salmon about 6 oz. each
- 4 tsp. Cajun seasoning
- 2 med. avocados, diced

Directions:

1. Heat a skillet over medium-high heat and warm the oil in it.
2. Rub the Cajun seasoning into the fillets, and then lay them into the bottom of the skillet once it's hot enough.

3. Cook until a dark crust forms, then flip and repeat.
4. In a medium mixing bowl, combine all the Ingredients: for the salsa and set aside.
5. Plate the fillets and top with 1/2of the salsa yielded.

BLT Salad

Ingredients:

- 6 bacon slices, cooked and chopped
- 2 hardboiled eggs, chopped
- 1 tablespoon roasted unsalted sunflower seeds
- 1 teaspoon toasted sesame seeds
- 1 cooked chicken breast, sliced optional
- 2 tablespoons melted bacon fat
- 2 tablespoons red wine vinegar
- Freshly ground black pepper
- 4 cups shredded lettuce
- 1 tomato, chopped

Directions:

1. In a medium bowl, whisk together the bacon fat and vinegar until emulsified.

2. Season with black pepper.
3. Add the tomato and lettuce to the bowl and toss the vegetables with the dressing.
4. Divide the salad between 4 plates and top each with equal amounts of bacon, egg, sunflower seeds, sesame seeds, and chicken if using. Serve.

Crab-stuffed Avocado

Ingredients:

- 1/2cup chopped, peeled English cucumber
- 1scallion, chopped
- 1 teaspoon chopped cilantro
- Pinch sea salt
- Freshly ground black pepper
- 1 avocado, peeled, halved lengthwise, and pitted
- 1teaspoon freshly squeezed lemon juice
- 41ounces Dungeness crabmeat
- 1cup cream cheese
- 1/2cup chopped red bell pepper

Directions:

1. Brush the cut edges of the avocado with the lemon juice and set the halves aside on a plate.
2. In a bowl or container, the crabmeat, cream cheese, red pepper, cucumber, scallion, cilantro, salt, and pepper must be well mixed.
3. The crab mixture will then be divided between the avocado

Grilled Halloumi Cheese with Eggs

Ingredients:

- 6 eggs, beaten
- 1tsp. sea salt
- 1/2tsp. crushed red pepper flakes
- 1 1cups avocado, pitted and sliced
- 1 cup grape tomatoes, halved
- 4 tbsp. pecans, chopped
- 4 slices halloumi cheese
- 3 tsp. olive oil
- 1 tsp. dried Greek seasoning blend
- 1 tbsp. olive oil

Directions:

1. Preheat your grill to medium.
2. Set the Halloumi in the center of a piece of heavy-duty foil.

3. Sprinkle oil over the Halloumi and apply Greek seasoning blend.
4. Close the foil to create a packet.
5. Grill for about 15 minutes, and then slice into four pieces.
6. In a frying pan, warm one tablespoon of oil and cook the eggs.
7. Stir well to create large and soft curds—season with salt and pepper.
8. Put the eggs and grilled cheese on a serving bowl.
9. Serve alongside tomatoes and avocado, decorated with chopped pecans.

Creamy Kale Salad

Ingredients:

- 1 bunch spinach
- 1 1tablespoon lemon juice
- 1 cup sour cream
- 1 cup roasted macadamia
- 2 tablespoons sesame seeds oil
- 1 1garlic clove, minced
- 1teaspoon black pepper
- 1/2teaspoon salt
- 2 tablespoons lime juice
- 1 bunch kale
- Toppings:
- 1 1Avocado, diced
- 1/2cup Pecans, chopped

Directions:

1. First of all, please confirm you've all the Ingredients: out there.
2. Chop kale and wash kale then remove the ribs.
3. Now transfer kale to a large bowl.
4. One thing remains to be done.
5. Add sour cream, lime juice, macadamia, sesame seeds oil, pepper, salt, garlic.
6. Finally, mix thoroughly.
7. Top with your avocado and pecans.
8. Serve& enjoy.

More Keto Recipes

Ingredients:

- 1 teaspoon of cinnamon

- 2 eggs

- 2 ounces of cream cheese

- 1to 1 packet of Stevia

- 1 tablespoon of coconut flour

Directions:

1. Combine well all of the Ingredients: in a bowl until the mixture is smooth, then heat a skillet over medium to high heat and add in coconut oil.
2. Add a scoop of the batter into the heated pan and cook for about 2 minutes on both sides.
3. Repeat the same for the remaining batter.
4. Top the pancakes with sugar free maple syrup.

Greek Style Lamb Chops

Ingredients:

- 2 tablespoons lemon juice
- 2 teaspoon oil
- 2 teaspoon salt
- 8 pcs of lamb loin chops, around 4 ounces
- 1 tablespoon black pepper
- 1 tablespoon dried oregano
- 1 tablespoon minced garlic

Directions:

1. In a big bowl or dish, combine the black pepper, salt, minced garlic, lemon juice and oregano.
2. Then rub it equally on all sides of the lamb chops.
3. Then place a skillet on high heat.

4. After a minute, coat skillet with the cooking spray and place the lamb chops.
5. Sear the lamb chops for a minute on each side.
6. Lower heat to medium; continue cooking lamb chops for 2-3 minutes per side or until desired doneness is reached.
7. Let it cool.

Bacon-Wrapped Roasted Asparagus

Ingredients:

- 16 asparagus spear, ends trimmed
- 16 pieces of bacon
- 2 tablespoons extra-virgin olive oil
- Salt and pepper to taste

Directions:

1. Preheat the oven to 4000F.
2. Line a baking sheet with aluminum foil or parchment paper.
3. Place the dry asparagus and place it on the baking sheet.
4. Drizzle with olive oil and toss to coat. Add salt and pepper to taste.
5. Wrap each spear with the bacon. Bake for 10 more minutes. Let it cool.

Keto Reuben Skillet

Ingredients:

- 9 ounces of drained sauerkraut

- 10 ounces of corned beef

- 2 tablespoons of butter

- 1 dill pickle

- 4 ounces of Swiss cheese

- 1 cup of mayonnaise

- 1 tablespoon of Dijon mustard

Directions:

1. Put some butter in a skillet on medium to low heat.
2. Put in beef and carefully fry it, then dry the sauerkraut.
3. Remove as much liquid from it and place evenly in a skillet.

4. Put some scoops of mustard in the skillet with the sauerkraut, then put in Swiss cheese and cook until the cheese begins to melt.
5. Cover the pan to make the mixture to cook faster.
6. Serve with more mustard and dill pickles.

Cauli Mac and Cheese

Ingredients:

- 1 cup cream cheese
- 1 teaspoon turmeric powder
- 1 teaspoon garlic paste
- 1 teaspoon onion flakes
- 1 head cauliflower, cut into florets
- 2 tablespoons ghee, melted
- Salt and black pepper, to taste
- 1 cup crème fraîche
- 1 cup half-and-half

Directions:

1. Set oven to 450ºF. Grease a baking sheet with cooking spray.
2. Shake cauliflower florets with melted ghee, salt, and pepper.

3. Arrange on the baking sheet and roast for 15 minutes. In a saucepan over medium heat, pour the remaining Ingredients: and heat through, stirring frequently.
4. Reduce heat to low and simmer for 2-3 minutes until thickened.
5. Coat the cauliflower florets in the cheese sauce and serve immediately in serving bowls.

Cheese & Pumpkin Chicken Meatballs

Ingredients:

- 1 onion, chopped
- 1 tablespoon Italian mixed herbs
- Salt and black pepper, to taste
- 2 tablespoon olive oil
- 1 cup cheddar cheese, shredded
- 1 egg, beaten
- 1 pound ground chicken
- 1 carrot, grated
- 2 garlic cloves, minced

Directions:

1. Set oven to 360ºF. Combine all Ingredients:, excluding cheese.
2. Form meatballs from the mixture; set them on a parchment-lined baking sheet.
3. Bake for 25 minutes, flipping once.

4. Spread cheese over the balls and bake for 7 more minutes or until all cheese melts.

Cheese, Ham and Egg Muffins

Ingredients:

- 1cup fresh parsley, chopped
- 1cup ricotta cheese
- 1cup Brie, chopped
- 24 slices smoked ham
- 6 eggs, beaten
- Salt and black pepper, to taste

Directions:

1. Set oven to 390ºF.
2. Line 2 slices of smoked ham to each muffin cup to circle each mold.
3. In a mixing bowl, mix the rest of the Ingredients:.
4. Fill 2 of the ham lined muffin cup with the egg/cheese mixture.
5. Bake for 15 minutes. Serve warm.

Beef and Kale Pan

Ingredients:

- 1 red onion, chopped
- 2 garlic cloves, minced
- 1 cup beef stock
- 1 teaspoon sweet paprika
- 1 tablespoon cilantro, chopped
- 1 pound beef stew meat, cubed
- 1 tablespoon olive oil
- 1 cup kale, torn
- 1 teaspoon chili powder
- 1 teaspoon rosemary, dried

Directions:

1. Ensure that you heat the pan; add the onion and the garlic, stir and sauté for 2 minutes.
2. Add the meat and brown it for 5 minutes.

3. Add the rest of the Ingredients:, bring to a simmer then cook over medium heat for 13 minutes more.
4. Divide the mix between plates and serve for lunch.

Chili Egg Pickles

Ingredients:

- 1 teaspoon yellow seeds
- 2 cloves garlic, sliced
- 1 cup vinegar
- 1cups water
- 1 tablespoon salt
- 10 eggs
- 1 cup onions, sliced
- 3 cardamom pods
- 1 tablespoon chili powder

Directions:

1. Boil eggs in salted water until hard-cooked, about 10 minutes; rinse under cold, running water; peel and discard the shell.
2. Place the peeled eggs into a large jar. Set a pan over medium heat.

3. Stir in all remaining Ingredients:; bring to a rapid boil.
4. Reduce heat to low; allow simmering for 6 minutes.
5. Spoon this mixture into the jar. Refrigerate for 2 to 3 weeks.

Gingery Tuna Mousse

Ingredients:

- 1/4 teaspoon ginger, grated
- 3 tablespoons water
- 3 tablespoons mayonnaise
- 3 ounces canned tuna, flaked
- 1 garlic clove, minced
- 1teaspoon black pepper
- 2 teaspoon gelatin, powdered
- 2 ounces ricotta cheese
- 1 teaspoon mustard
- 1cup onions, chopped
- 1 teaspoon salt

Directions:

1. Mix gelatin in water; let sit for 10 minutes.

2. Set a pan over medium heat and warm ricotta cheese; place in gelatin and mix to blend well; let the mixture cool.
3. Place in the other Ingredients: and stir.
4. Split the mixture among 5 mousse molds and refrigerate overnight.
5. Serve by inverting the molds over a serving platter.

Creamy Cheddar Deviled Eggs

Ingredients:

- 2 tablespoons carrot, chopped
- 2 tablespoons chives, minced
- 2 tablespoons cheddar cheese, grated
- Salt and black pepper, to taste
- 10 eggs
- 1cup mayonnaise
- 1 tablespoon tomato paste
- 2 tablespoons celery, chopped

Directions:

1. Place the eggs in a pot and fill with water by about 1 inch.
2. Bring the eggs to a boil over high heat, then reduce the heat to medium and simmer for 10 minutes.

3. Remove and rinse under running water until cooled. Peel and discard the shell.
4. Slice each egg in half lengthwise and get rid of the yolks.
5. Mix the yolks with the rest of the Ingredients:.
6. Split the mixture amongst the egg whites and set deviled eggs on a plate to serve.

Pan-fried vegetables with avocado dip

Ingredients:

- 120 g zucchini
- 120 g cauliflower
- 120 g broccoli
- salt
- curry
- 1 tbsp coconut oil
- 1 /2 Avocado
- 1 squirt of lemon juice
- black pepper, ground

Directions:

1. Wash, clean and cut the vegetables.
2. Fry in the coconut oil in a pan and season with salt, pepper and curry powder.
3. Then remove the avocado from the peel, puree with lemon, salt, pepper and a little

water or mash with a fork until a creamy dip is obtained.
4. Serve both together.

Lasagne

Ingredients:

- 1 small clove of garlic
- Some rosemary
- Chili powder
- Paprika powder
- salt and pepper
- Oil for thickening
- 120 g lasagne platters zucchini slices or konjac platters
- 320 g chopped tomatoes from the can
- 170 g natural tofu
- 1-2 tbsp tomato paste
- 190 g spinach leaves
- 240 ml soy milk unsweetened

Directions:

1. Cut the onion and the clove of garlic into small pieces and fry them in the pan with oil.
2. The water from the tofu with paper towels to absorb and cut into small pieces after.
3. Now fry the tofu in the pan for at least 8 minutes.
4. Season the tofu slices with pepper, sea salt, paprika powder and chili powder.
5. Add the chopped canned tomatoes.
6. Also add a little rosemary to the sauce.
7. Now blanch the spinach in hot water for at least 8 minutes.
8. Then rinse the spinach with cold water. Season the spinach to taste.
9. Now layer the Ingredients: in the baking dish. Start with the tofu mixture.
10. Then come the lasagna platters. The layering must end with the tofu mixture.

11. The lasagna must then be put in the oven for at least half an hour at 200 degrees.

Italian Vegetable Pan

Ingredients:

- 40 g pine nuts
- 1 clove of garlic
- 140 g mushrooms
- Sea salt and pepper
- 220 g spinach
- half an onion
- 1 sprig of oregano
- 1tbsp coconut oil

Directions:

1. First clean the spinach and let it drain.
2. Wash the oregano as well then remove the leaves from the stem.
3. Wash the mushrooms and then trim them into small pieces.

4. Peel the onion and cut into small cubes. Peel the garlic clove and then finely chop it.
5. Sprinkle the garlic with a little salt. Put the coconut oil in a pan.
6. Then add the onion pieces and garlic pieces to the pan.
7. Add pine nuts. Season the Ingredients: as desired .
8. After a few minutes add the spinach, mushrooms and oregano.
9. Fry everything for 10 minutes and then season again with pepper and salt.

Kohlrabi fries

Ingredients:

- 1 tbsp paprika powder
- 1 tbsp olive oil
- rosemary
- a large kohlrabi
- pepper salt

Directions:

1. At the beginning preheat the oven to 180 degrees.
2. Peel the kohlrabi and cut into fries-shaped pieces.
3. Put the oil, paprika and pepper in a freezer bag.
4. Add the kohlrabi fries and mix everything together well.
5. Cover a baking sheet with parchment paper and then spread the kohlrabi fries on it.

6. Let the fries stew in the oven for half an hour.
7. Sprinkle the French fries with salt at the end.

Coconut Thai curry

Ingredients:

- 270 g broccoli
- 1 zucchini
- 1 bell pepper
- 1cup pineapple
- 1cup mango
- 90 g bamboo shoots
- Chili powder
- half an eggplant
- 1 carrot
- 1 tbsp curry powder
- 1 tbsp curry paste
- half an onion
- 220 g coconut milk
- Sea salt and pepper

Directions:

1. First, let the broccoli simmer for 6 minutes.
2. Cut the fruit into small cubes.
3. Cut the remaining vegetables into equally sized slices.
4. Fry the vegetables and fruits in a little oil for 8 minutes.
5. Season the Ingredients: in between .
6. Now add the bamboo shoots and stir in
7. Now simmer for another 10 minutes and at the end season with curry powder, curry, salt and pepper.

Savoy cabbage stew

Ingredients:

- 70 ml coconut milk
- half a red chilli pepper
- a stick of lemongrass
- 2 tbsp lemon juice
- 1 teaspoon vegetable stock
- Pepper and sea salt
- 140 g savoy cabbage
- 220 g carrots
- 220 g celery
- 1 a teaspoon of coconut oil
- 1 a bunch of spring onions

Directions:

1. Wash the cabbage and cut into fine pieces with the kitchen knife.

2. Then clean the parsnips and carrots and cut into fine sticks.
3. Cut the onions into rings of the same size .
4. Repeat the same with the lemongrass.
5. Now cut the red chilli in half and heat the coconut oil in a saucepan.
6. Steam the onions in the pan until translucent.
7. After a few minutes add the honey and mix with the onions.
8. Spices can also be added at this point.
9. Now put the kale in the pot and simmer for another 2 minutes.
10. Season with salt and pepper.
11. Add parsnips and carrots to the pan and simmer.
12. Stir in the lemongrass. Then add the water. Then mix in a little salt.
13. Let the stew simmer over medium heat for 15 minutes.

14. After 5 minutes, add the coconut milk and the chili halves to the saucepan.
15. Then season to taste with salt, lemon juice and pepper.

Pizza with fresh vegetables

Ingredients:

- 1 tbsp Italian herbs
- 120 g tomatoes
- 1 chili pepper
- 2 tbsp olive oil
- Salt and pepper
- 120 g of shredded mozzarella
- 40 g tomato paste
- 80 g mushrooms
- 1 eggplant

Directions:
1. First preheat the oven to 180 degrees.
2. Cut the aubergine into slices and season with salt.
3. Cook the aubergine in the oven for 10 minutes.

4. Then mix the tomato paste with the spices and olive oil.
5. Pour the mixture on the eggplants.
6. Cut the mozzarella, tomatoes, chili pepper and mushrooms into small pieces and distribute them on the aubergine.
7. Bake the whole thing in the oven for another 10 minutes. Then serve.

Vegan keto pizza

Ingredients:

For the ground:

- 1/4 cup hot water
- a bit of salt
- 60 g of flaxseed
- 1/2tbsp garlic powder

For covering:

- 2 tbsp dried tomatoes
- vegan cheese / vegan feta optional
- Sea salt and pepper
- 2 olives
- 1/2cup pesto

Directions:

1. First preheat the oven to 180 degrees circulating air.

2. Then slowly stir the flax seeds into the hot water.
3. A bowl should be used for this, as the garlic powder and salt must be added immediately afterwards.
4. So l until it forms a paste is stirred. This step can take a few minutes.
5. Once a dough is formed, it must be divided into two different parts.
6. Now knead two balls of the same size out of the dough.
7. Put the oil in a non-stick pan and heat over medium heat.
8. Place a ball of dough in the center of the pan. Flatten the dough ball.
9. Turn the dough over and fry for 1 minute on each side.
10. Repeat this process with the second dough ball .
11. Cover the dough with the Ingredients:.

12. Finally, put the pizza in the preheated oven 180 degrees for 10 minutes.

Cauliflower pizza with salami

Ingredients:

- 30 g almond flour
- 1teaspoon psyllium husks
- 2 tbsp olive oil
- Italian herbs
- salt and pepper
- 1 whole cauliflower
- 120 g parmesan
- 50g canned tomatoes chopped
- 120 g grated cheese e.g. Emmentaler
- 70 g salami
- 1 egg

Directions:

1. Split the cauliflower, cut off the florets, put in a blender and chop until a fine powder is formed.
2. Put the cauliflower powder in a microwave-safe container and cook covered for 4 minutes on the highest level.
3. Then place on a kitchen towel and let cool down well.
4. The steamed cauliflower must be thoroughly squeezed out with the kitchen towel until no excess liquid comes out.
5. Mix the Parmesan, 30g of the Emmentaler, psyllium husks and the almond flour in a bowl.
6. Then add the cauliflower and the egg, as dry as possible.
7. Mix the mixture with a spoon or your hands and season with salt, pepper and the Italian herbs.

8. The dough is now spread on a baking sheet lined with baking paper, pressed firmly and pushed into the oven for 15-20 minutes at 220 degrees until the dough is light golden brown.
9. For the topping, distribute the chopped canned tomatoes on the dough and season with Italian herbs, salt and pepper.
10. Spread the rest of the Emmentaler cheese and salami on the dough as well.
11. Now the pizza comes back into the oven for about 10 minutes until the cheese has melted. Finally pour the olive oil over it.

Pizza with cheese base

Ingredients:

- 20 g olives
- 30 g salami
- 40 g cheese
- 2 egg
- 90 g mozzarella
- 30 g tomato paste

Directions:

1. First mix the eggs with the mozzarella and place the batter on a baking sheet.
2. Bake for 15 minutes at 200 degrees in the preheated oven until the dough is golden brown.
3. Then let it cool down briefly.
4. Spread the tomato paste on the pizza base and top with the remaining Ingredients:.

5. Bake at 220 degrees for 5-10 minutes until the cheese has melted and is crispy brown.

Crunchy salami pizza

Ingredients:

- 1 teaspoon cream cheese
- 1 teaspoon apple cider vinegar
- 140 g canned tomatoes strained
- Italian herbs
- 520 g grated mozzarella
- 200 g almond flour
- 1 egg
- 1teaspoon salt
- olive oil
- 220 g salami

Directions:

1. First preheat the oven to 200 degrees and line a baking sheet with parchment paper.

2. Put 300g of grated mozzarella with 2 teaspoons of cream cheese in a non-stick coated pan and heat until both can be mixed.
3. Optionally, the mozzarella and cream cheese can also be put in the microwave and melted there.
4. Add the almond flour, egg, vinegar and salt and mix the Ingredients: together until a batter is formed.
5. Now place the dough on the baking sheet and form a circle with a diameter of approx. 20 cm.
6. Prick the dough all over with a fork.
7. Then put the dough in the oven for 10-12 minutes , until it is golden brown.
8. Take the dough out of the oven and brush with a thin layer of tomato puree.
9. Sprinkle the cheese on top and top the pizza with salami.
10. Finally, pour a pinch of Italian herbs on top.

11. Finally, bake the pizza again in the oven for 10-15 minutes until the cheese melts and the salami is a little crispy.

Pizza Margherita

Ingredients:

For the dough:

- 70 g of pureed tomatoes
- 20 g coconut flour
- 120 g mozzarella
- 5 g psyllium husks
- 10 g chia seeds
- 80 ml of water
- 50 g flaxseed flour
- 120 g tomatoes
- 40 g almond flour

For covering:

- 20 g rocket
- 1 teaspoon dried basil
- salt and pepper

Directions:

1. Preheat the oven to 180 degrees circulating air
2. Mix the flax seeds with the almond flour, coconut flour, chia seeds, as well as flea seeds and salt.
3. Then add the water and stir. Let the dough rest in the refrigerator for 1 hour.
4. Shape the dough into small balls.
5. Put these on a baking sheet and roll out.
6. Bake the dough for 10 minutes. Cut the tomatoes and mozzarella into slices.
7. Spread the tomato sauce on the pizza bases. Season this with salt and pepper and spread the mozzarella on top.
8. Top the pizza with the rocket and sprinkle with the basil.

Avocado lime salmon

Ingredients:

- 2 tablespoons diced red onion
- 2 tablespoons olive oil
- 2 6-ounce boneless salmon fillets
- Salt and pepper
- 100 grams chopped cauliflower
- 1 large avocado
- 1 tablespoon fresh lime juice

Directions:

1. Place the cauliflower in a food processor and pulse into rice-like grains.
2. Grease a skillet with cooking spray and heat over medium heat.
3. Add the cauliflower rice and cook, covered, for 8 minutes until tender. Set aside.

4. Combine the avocado, lime juice and red onion in a food processor and blend smooth.
5. Heat the oil in a large skillet over medium-high heat.
6. Season the salmon with salt and pepper then add to the skillet skin-side down.
7. Cook for 4 to 5 minutes until seared then flip and cook for another 4 to 5 minutes.
8. Serve the salmon over a bed of cauliflower rice topped with the avocado cream. Makes 2 servings.

Rosemary roasted chicken and veggies

Ingredients:

- 1 small parsnip, peeled and sliced
- 2 cloves garlic, sliced
- 3 tablespoons olive oil
- 1 tablespoon balsamic vinegar
- 2 teaspoons fresh chopped rosemary
- 4 deboned chicken thighs
- Salt and pepper
- 1 small zucchini, sliced
- 2 small carrots, peeled and sliced

Directions:

1. Preheat the oven to 350°F and lightly grease a small rimmed baking sheet with cooking spray.

2. Place the chicken thighs on the baking sheet and season with salt and pepper.
3. Arrange the veggies around the chicken then sprinkle with sliced garlic.
4. Whisk together the remaining Ingredients: then drizzle over the chicken and veggies.
5. Bake for 30 minutes then broil for 3 to 5 minutes until the skins are crisp. Makes 2 servings.

Cheesy Sausage and Mushroom Skillet

Ingredients:

- 1 small yellow onion, chopped
- 1 teaspoon dried oregano
- 1/2 teaspoon dried thyme
- Salt and pepper
- 1/2 cup marinara sauce
- 1/2 cup water
- 1 cup shredded mozzarella cheese
- 1 tablespoon coconut oil
- 6 ounces Italian sausage, crumbled
- 4 ounces sliced mushrooms

Directions:

1. Preheat the oven to 350°F.
2. Heat the oil in a large cast-iron skillet over medium heat until smoking.

3. Add the sausages and cook until browned and almost cooked through.
4. Remove the sausages to a cutting board and let cool for a few minutes.
5. Add the mushroom and onion to the skillet and cook for 3 to 4 minutes until browned.
6. Slice the sausages and add them back to the skillet.
7. Stir in the oregano, thyme, salt and pepper.
8. Pour in the sauce and water then stir well. Transfer the skillet to the oven and cook for 10 minutes.
9. Sprinkle with mozzarella then cook for another 5 minutes until melted. Makes 2 servings.

Lamb Chops with Rosemary and Garlic

Ingredients:

- 2 bone-in lamb chops about 6 ounces meat
- 1 tablespoon butter
- Salt and pepper
- 1/2 pound fresh asparagus, trimmed
- 1 tablespoon olive oil
- 1 tablespoon coconut oil, melted
- 1 teaspoon fresh chopped rosemary
- 1 clove garlic, minced

Directions:

1. Combine the coconut oil, rosemary, and garlic in a shallow dish.
2. Add the lamb chops then turn to coat – let marinate in the fridge overnight.
3. Let the lamb rest at room temperature for 30 minutes.

4. Heat the butter in a large skillet over medium-high heat.
5. Add the lamb chops and cook for 6 minutes then season with salt and pepper.
6. Turn the chops and cook for another 6 minutes or until cooked to the desired level.
7. Let the lamb chops rest for 5 minutes before serving.
8. Meanwhile, toss the asparagus with olive oil, salt and pepper then spread on a baking sheet.
9. Broil for 6 to 8 minutes until charred, shaking occasionally. Serve hot with the lamb chops.

Keto Low-Carb Cheesy Tacos Skillet

Ingredients:

- Diced large Onion 1
- Sliced large Bell peppers 3
- 1 can of Diced tomatoes of 14.5 oz
- Mexican cheese blend 1 c
- Sliced Green onions 1/2 c
- Ground beef 1 lb.
- Taco seasoning 2 tbsp.
- Water 1 c

Directions:

1. Heat skillet over moderate to high heat.
2. Add the ground beef and cook for about ten minutes until browned, breaking the beef apart with a spatula or spoon.
3. Add water and taco seasoning.

4. Cook for two-three minutes until it absorbs or evaporates the excess water.
5. Reduce to medium heat.
6. Add the bell peppers and the onions.
7. Cook for 5-10 mins until the onions are translucent and soft.
8. Stir in the chopped tomatoes. Simmer for several minutes, until heat evaporates as well as any excess moisture.
9. Reduce to low heat.
10. Sprinkle over with shredded cheese.
11. Cover the pan and heat until the cheese has melted.
12. Remove the green onions from heat and top.

Keto Veggie & fruits smoothie

Ingredients:

- Ginger peeled 1 inch
- English cucumber peeled ¾
- Lemon peeled 1
- Frozen avocado 1 cup
- Coldwater 1 cup
- Baby spinach 1 cup
- Cilantro 1cup

Directions:

1. Apply all the components to the high-velocity blender and combine until smooth.
2. Place in the refrigerator in a sealed jar such as a mason jar for 3 days.

Keto Iced Caramel Macchiato

Ingredients:

- Torani sugar-free caramel syrup 1 cup
- Unsalted butter 1/2 cup
- Heavy whipping cream 1/2 cup

For serving

- Unsweetened almond milk 1 cup
- Ice 4 cups
- Coffee brewed strong 2 cups

For topping

- Torani sugar-free caramel syrup
- Whipped cream

Directions:

1. In a deep saucepan, unsalted butter & strong whipping cream combined on medium heat, stirring constantly.

2. Stir almost constantly until the creamer develops a light-yellow color and thickens sufficiently to brush a spoon's rim, around 4-5 minutes until the mix comes to boil.
3. Slowly add in the Torani sugar-free syrup and whisk well.
4. Let the mix cool down slowly.
5. Load up with ice on four bottles. Load 1/2cup of almond milk and 2 tsp of the creamer you've just made into the bottom of each bottle, then mix.
6. Pour espresso or a good coffee fast. Do not move.
7. Cover the sugar-free caramel sauce with whipped cream & drizzle over.
8. Serve in the bottom with creamer and sugar in the center with the coffee and top with whipped cream.

Peanut Butter Granola

Ingredients:

- Collagen protein powder or vanilla whey protein powder 1/4 cup
- Peanut butter 1/4 cup
- Butter 1/2cup
- Water 1/2cup
- Almonds 1 1cups
- Pecans 1 1cups
- Almond flour or shredded coconut 1 cup
- Sunflower seeds 1/2cup
- Swerve sweetener 1/4 cup

Directions:

1. Oven preheated to 300f & line a large baking paper with a covered baking tray.
2. In the mixing bowl, process the almonds and pecans with larger pieces until they resemble-

fine scraps. Mix in chopped nuts, sweeteners, sunflower seeds & vanilla whey protein and transfer it to the large bowl.

3. Evaporate peanut butter & butter together in a non - stick frying pan.
4. Place melted peanut butter over a mixture of nuts and mix excellently, tossing lightly.
5. Mix the mixture.
6. Combine clumps around each other.
7. Spread the mixture evenly over the ready baking sheet & bake for 30 mins, mixing through halfway.
8. Remove and allow it to cool.

Keto Salted Caramel Hot Chocolate

Ingredients:

- Salted caramel collagen 1-2 tbsp.
- Liquid or powdered sweetener
- optional whipped cream lightly sweetened
- optional caramel sauce sugar-free
- Hemp milk or unsweetened almond 1cup
- Heavy whipping cream 2 tablespoons
- Cocoa powder 1 tbsp.

Directions:

1. In a small saucepan over medium heat, combine the almond or hemp milk and the heavy cream.
2. Bring it to a simmer.
3. Add the cocoa powder and collagen to a blender.
4. Pour in the hot milk and blend until frothy.

5. Taste and adjust for sweetness.
6. Top with lightly sweetened whipped cream and some homemade caramel sauce to take it over the top.

Keto Brownie Bark

Ingredients:

- Cocoa powder 3 tbsp.
- Instant coffee optional 1 tsp
- Butter melted 1/2cup
- Heavy whipping cream 1 tbsp.
- Vanilla 1tsp
- Chocolate chips sugar-free 1/4 cups
- Almond flour 1cup
- Baking powder 1tsp
- Salt 1/2tsp
- Egg whites 2 large
- Swerve sweetener granular 1cup

Directions:

1. Oven preheated to 325f, and line a baking sheet with bakery release paper.
2. Greaseproof paper to the bakery release paper.
3. Stir together all the baking powder, almond powder, and salt in the small bowl.
4. Beat a white egg in the large mixing bowl until they're frothy.
5. Beat until smooth in cocoa powder, sweetener & instant coffee, after which beat in softened butter, vanilla & cream.
6. Beat in a mixture of almond meal until it's combined.
7. Spread batter over nonstick baking paper in a 12 by 8-inch rectangle.
8. Stir the chocolate morsels.
9. Bake and set for 18 mins until puffed.
10. Now remove it from the oven and turn off the Oven and allow to cool for 15 mins.

11. To cut it into 2inch squares, use a filet knife or pizza cutter but don't separate. Return it to a hot oven for 8-10 mins to gently crisp up.
12. Remove, allow it to cool down & then split it into squares.

Keto Pork Loin Roast with Herb Seasoning

Ingredients:

- Onion powder 2 tbsp.

- Italian herb seasoning 2 tbsp.

- Avocado oil 3 tbsp. 45 ml

- Boneless pork loin roast 3 lb.

- Garlic powder 1 tbsp.

- Salt & pepper >> to taste

Directions:

1. Preheat oven to 400 F 200 C and apply grease or cover an aluminum foil baking tray.
2. Attach the avocado oil over high heat to a frying pan.
3. Now use tongs to grill the pork loin and cook all over.

4. Alternatively, in a shallow pot, add the onion powder, garlic powder, black pepper, and Italian seasoning, oil.
5. Put the pork shoulder loin on the lined baking tray and spray or rub over the pork, the herb mixture be cautious, as it may still be hot. Bake for 35-45 mins in the oven.
6. Test the pork loin's internal temperature is at 145 F.
7. Remove from the oven, allow 10 minutes of rest to allow extra fluid to drain out, then slice and serve.

Lamb Chops with Rosemary and Garlic

Ingredients:

- 2 bone-in lamb chops about 6 ounces meat
- 1 tablespoon butter
- Salt and pepper
- 1/2 pound fresh asparagus, trimmed
- 1 tablespoon olive oil
- 1 tablespoon coconut oil, melted
- 1 teaspoon fresh chopped rosemary
- 1 clove garlic, minced

Directions:

1. Combine the coconut oil, rosemary, and garlic in a shallow dish.
2. Add the lamb chops then turn to coat – let marinate in the fridge overnight.
3. Let the lamb rest at room temperature for 30 minutes.

4. Heat the butter in a large skillet over medium-high heat.
5. Add the lamb chops and cook for 6 minutes then season with salt and pepper.
6. Turn the chops and cook for another 6 minutes or until cooked to the desired level.
7. Let the lamb chops rest for 5 minutes before serving.
8. Meanwhile, toss the asparagus with olive oil, salt and pepper then spread on a baking sheet.
9. Broil for 6 to 8 minutes until charred, shaking occasionally. Serve hot with the lamb chops.

Keto Low-Carb Cheesy Tacos Skillet

Ingredients:

- Diced large Onion 1
- Sliced large Bell peppers 3
- 1 can of Diced tomatoes of 14.5 oz
- Mexican cheese blend 1 c
- Sliced Green onions 1/2 c
- Ground beef 1 lb.
- Taco seasoning 2 tbsp.
- Water 1 c

Directions:
1. Heat skillet over moderate to high heat.
2. Add the ground beef and cook for about ten minutes until browned, breaking the beef apart with a spatula or spoon.
3. Add water and taco seasoning.

4. Cook for two-three minutes until it absorbs or evaporates the excess water.
5. Reduce to medium heat.
6. Add the bell peppers and the onions.
7. Cook for 5-10 mins until the onions are translucent and soft.
8. Stir in the chopped tomatoes. Simmer for several minutes, until heat evaporates as well as any excess moisture.
9. Reduce to low heat.
10. Sprinkle over with shredded cheese.
11. Cover the pan and heat until the cheese has melted.
12. Remove the green onions from heat and top.

Keto Veggie & fruits smoothie

Ingredients:

- Ginger peeled 1 inch
- English cucumber peeled ¾
- Lemon peeled 1
- Frozen avocado 1 cup
- Coldwater 1 cup
- Baby spinach 1 cup
- Cilantro 1cup

Directions:

1. Apply all the components to the high-velocity blender and combine until smooth.
2. Place in the refrigerator in a sealed jar such as a mason jar for 3 days.

Keto Iced Caramel Macchiato

Ingredients:

- Torani sugar-free caramel syrup 1 cup

- Unsalted butter 1/2 cup

- Heavy whipping cream 1/2 cup

For serving

- Unsweetened almond milk 1 cup

- Ice 4 cups

- Coffee brewed strong 2 cups

For topping

- Torani sugar-free caramel syrup

- Whipped cream

Directions:

1. In a deep saucepan, unsalted butter & strong whipping cream combined on medium heat, stirring constantly.

2. Stir almost constantly until the creamer develops a light-yellow color and thickens sufficiently to brush a spoon's rim, around 4-5 minutes until the mix comes to boil.
3. Slowly add in the Torani sugar-free syrup and whisk well.
4. Let the mix cool down slowly.
5. Load up with ice on four bottles. Load 1/2cup of almond milk and 2 tsp of the creamer you've just made into the bottom of each bottle, then mix.
6. Pour espresso or a good coffee fast. Do not move.
7. Cover the sugar-free caramel sauce with whipped cream & drizzle over.
8. Serve in the bottom with creamer and sugar in the center with the coffee and top with whipped cream.

Peanut Butter Granola

Ingredients:

- Collagen protein powder or vanilla whey protein powder 1/4 cup
- Peanut butter 1/4 cup
- Butter 1/2cup
- Water 1/2cup
- Almonds 1 1cups
- Pecans 1 1cups
- Almond flour or shredded coconut 1 cup
- Sunflower seeds 1/2cup
- Swerve sweetener 1/4 cup

Directions:

1. Oven preheated to 300f & line a large baking paper with a covered baking tray.
2. In the mixing bowl, process the almonds and pecans with larger pieces until they resemble-

fine scraps. Mix in chopped nuts, sweeteners, sunflower seeds & vanilla whey protein and transfer it to the large bowl.
3. Evaporate peanut butter & butter together in a non - stick frying pan.
4. Place melted peanut butter over a mixture of nuts and mix excellently, tossing lightly.
5. Mix the mixture.
6. Combine clumps around each other.
7. Spread the mixture evenly over the ready baking sheet & bake for 30 mins, mixing through halfway.
8. Remove and allow it to cool.

Keto Creamy Sun-Dried Tomato Chicken Thighs

Ingredients:

- 1 cup drained sun-dried tomatoes, chopped
- 4 cloves garlic, minced
- 1 tbsp Italian seasoning
- 1 cup heavy whipping cream
- 1/2 cup Parmesan cheese
- Chicken Thighs
- 1 cup grated Parmesan cheese
- 1.3pounds 6-pieces chicken thighs, skinless and boneless Salt and pepper, to taste
- Creamy Sauce
- 1/2 cup oil from jarred sun-dried tomatoes

Directions:

1. Combine the Parmesan cheese, salt, and some pepper in a plate.
2. Coat the chicken in the mixture to evenly.
3. Heat the sun-dried tomato oil in a large skillet over medium-high heat.
4. Sear the coated chicken for a fewminutes on each side, until browned. Set the seared chicken aside.
5. Place the sun-dried tomatoes, garlic, and Italian seasoning in the skillet and cook for a few minutes until thetomatoes start to soften.
6. Pour in the heavy cream and the remaining Parmesan cheese.
7. Combine to create the finished sauce.
8. Add the seared chicken back to the skillet and cook until the chicken cooked through.

Keto Ground Beef Stroganoff

Ingredients:

- 1 cup sour cream
- 1 tsp paprika
- 1 tbsp fresh lemon juice
- 1 tbsp fresh chopped parsley
- 2 tbsp butter
- 1 clove minced garlic
- 1 pound 80% lean ground beef
- Salt and pepper, to taste
- 10 oz228g sliced mushrooms
- 2 tbsp water

Directions:

1. In a large skillet over medium heat, add the butter.

2. When the butter has melted and stops foaming, add theminced garlic to the skillet.
3. Cook the garlic until fragrant, then mix in the ground beef—season with salt and pepper.
4. Cook the ground beef until no longer pink; break up the grounds with a wooden spoon.
5. Remove the cookedbeef from the skillet and transfer to a bowl and set aside.
6. Wipe most of the fat from the skillet, leaving just a little on the bottom to cook the mushrooms.
7. Add the mushrooms and water to the pan and cook over medium heat.
8. Cook until the liquid has reducedhalfway, and the mushrooms are tender.
9. Set the cooked mushrooms aside.
10. Reduce the heat then whisk the sour cream and paprika into the skillet.
11. Stir in the cooked beef and mushrooms into the pan and combine.

12. Stir in the lemon juice and parsley.

Pork and Mushroom Bake

Ingredients:

- 6 pork chops
- 1 cup sliced mushrooms
- Salt and ground pepper, to taste
- 1 onion, chopped
- 2 cans of mushroom soup

Directions:

1. Preheat the oven to 370ºF.
2. Spice the pork chops with salt and black pepper, and place in a baking dish.
3. Combine the mushroom soup, mushrooms, and onion, in a bowl.
4. Pour this mixture over the pork chops.
5. Bake for 45 minutes. Serve. Enjoy.

Juicy Pork Medallions

Ingredients:

- 1 cup vegetable stock

- Salt and black pepper, to taste

- 1-pound pork tenderloin, cut into medallions

- 2 onions, chopped

- 6 bacon slices, chopped

Directions:

1. Set a pan over medium heat, stir in the bacon, cook until crispy, and remove in a plate.
2. Add onions, black pepper, and salt, and cook for 5 minutes; set to the same plate with bacon.
3. Add the pork medallions to the pan, season with black pepper and salt, brown for 3 minutes on each side, turn, reduce heat to medium, and cook for 7 minutes.
4. Stir in the stock, and cook for 2 minutes.

5. Return the bacon and onions to the pan and cook for 1 minute. Serve when done.

Pulled Pork with Avocado

Ingredients:

- 1 cup vegetable stock
- 1/2 cup jerk seasoning
- 6 avocadoes, sliced
- 4 pounds of pork shoulder
- 1 tablespoon avocado oil

Directions:

1. Rub the pork shoulder with jerk seasoning, and set in a greased baking dish.
2. Pour in the stock, and cook for 1 hour 45 minutes in the oven at 350ºF covered with aluminum foil.
3. Discard the foil and cook for another 20 minutes.
4. Leave to rest for 30 minutes, and shred it with 2 forks.
5. Serve topped with avocado slices.

Buffalo Shrimp Lettuce Wraps

Ingredients:

- For 1 lb. Peeled and deveined shrimp, tails cut.
- Salt of Kosher
- Black pepper freshly roasted
- 1 Romaine head, different leaves, for serving
- 2 Red onion, thinly chopped
- 1 Rib Celery, thinly sliced
- 1/2 of a c. Crumbled blue cheese
- With 1/4 tbsp. Butter
- 2 Cloves of garlic, minced
- 1/4 of a c. Hot sauce, for example, Frank's
- For 1 tbsp Olive Oil Extra-Virgin

Directions:

1. Create the buffalo sauce: Melt the butter in a small saucepan over medium heat.
2. When fully melted, add garlic and simmer for 1 minute, until fragrant.

3. To mix, add hot sauce and stir. Switch the heat to low while the shrimp is frying.
4. Create shrimp: Heat oil in a large skillet over medium heat.
5. Attach the shrimp and season with pepper and salt.
6. Cook, turning halfway, until both sides are pink and invisible, around 2 minutes on either side.
7. Turn the fire off, apply the buffalo sauce and toss to coat.
8. Add to the middle of the Romaine leaf a little scoop of shrimp.
9. Then finish with red onion, celery.
10. Blue cheese.

Keto Bacon Sushi

Ingredients:

- 1 Sliced avocado
- 4 of an oz. Cream cheese softened, softened.
- Seeds of sesame for garnish.
- 6 bacon strips, halved
- 2 Persian cucumbers, cut thinly
- 2 Thinly diced, medium carrots.

Directions:

1. Preheat the oven to 400 degrees. Line a baking sheet and match it with a cooling rack with aluminum foil.
2. Lay bacon halves in an even layer and bake for 11 to 13 minutes until mildly crisp but still pliable.
3. Meanwhile, cut approximately the width of the bacon into pieces of cucumbers, carrots, and avocado.

4. Spread an equal layer of cream cheese on each slice until the bacon is cold enough to touch it.
5. Divide the vegetables into the bacon equally and put them on one end.
6. Strictly roll up the vegetables.
7. Garnish with and serve the sesame seeds.

Keto Burger Fat Bombs

Ingredients:

- For 2 tbsp. Cold butter, 20 bits of sliced butter
- Of 2 oz. Split into 20 bits of Cheddar,
- Leaves of spinach, to be eaten
- Tomatoes, thinly cut, for serving
- Mustard, to be eaten
- Spray for cooking For 1 lb.
- Ground-based cattle Of 1/2 tsp.
- Powdered garlic
- Salt of Kosher
- Black pepper freshly roasted

Directions:

1. Preheat the oven to 375 °C and oil the cooking spray with a mini muffin tin.
2. Season the beef with garlic powder, salt, and pepper in a medium dish.

3. Push 1 teaspoon of beef equally, covering the bottom entirely, into the bottom of each muffin tin cup.
4. Place a piece of butter on top and press 1 teaspoon of meat over the butter to cover full.
5. In each cup, place a slice of Cheddar on top of the meat and force the remaining beef over the cheese to cover it fully.
6. Bake for about 15 minutes before the meat is ready. Let yourself cool somewhat.
7. Using a metal offset spatula carefully to release each burger out of the tin.
8. Serve with onions, salad leaves, and mustard.

Keto Taco Cups

Ingredients:

- Of 1/2 tsp. Tweet Paprika
- Salt of Kosher
- Black pepper freshly roasted
- For serving sour cream,
- Diced avocado, to be eaten
- Cilantro, finely chopped, for serving.
- Tomatoes, diced, for serving
- 2 c. Cheddar Shredded
- For 1 tbsp. Olive Oil Extra-Virgin
- 1 Micro onion, chopped.
- 3 Garlic cloves, minced
- For 1 lb. Ground-based cattle
- For 1 tsp. Powdered chili
- Of 1/2 tsp. Cumin from the ground

Directions:

1. Preheat the oven to 375 ° and use parchment paper to cover a large baking sheet.

2. Spoon 2 teaspoons of Cheddar a couple of inches apart.
3. Bake for about 6 minutes, until bubbly and the edges tend to turn golden.
4. Enable the baking sheet to cool for a minute.
5. Meanwhile, oil the muffin tin bottom with a cooking spray, gently pick up the slices of melted cheese and put them on the bottom.
6. Add another inverted muffin tin and allow to cool for 10 minutes.
7. Using your hands helps mold the cheese around the inverted pan because you do not have a second muffin tin.
8. Heat the oil in a big skillet over medium heat.
9. Attach the onion and simmer for about 5 minutes, stirring periodically, until tender.
10. Stir in the garlic, then apply the ground beef and a wooden spoon to break up the pork.
11. Cook for about 6 minutes, until the beef is no longer pink, then remove the fat.

12. Put the meat back in the pan and season with chili powder, cumin, salt, pepper and paprika.
13. Move the cups of cheese into a serving bowl.
14. Cover it with cooked ground beef and top it with sour cream, cilantro, avocado, and tomatoes.

Shrimp salad with yogurt dressing

Ingredients:

- 2 tablespoons of natural yogurt
- 1 squirt of lemon juice
- 1 teaspoon sesame
- 100 g cherry tomatoes
- 1 handful of baby spinach
- 2 teaspoons olive oil
- 120 g prawns
- salt
- pepper

Directions:

1. First of all, cut the tomatoes in half and put them on a plate along with the spinach .
2. Now heat the teaspoon of olive oil in a pan and stir-fry the prawns for 3 minutes.

3. The prawns can be seasoned with salt and pepper to taste.
4. To make the dressing, the yogurt must be mixed with 1 tablespoon of olive oil, lemon juice and a little salt and pepper.
5. Garnish the prawns on the salad.

Keto Kale & Sausage Soup

Ingredients:
- 1/2 teaspoon of Crushed Red Pepper Flakes
- 1 cup of Heavy Whipping Cream
- 4 cups of Low-Sodium Chicken Broth
- 3 cups of Chopped Kale
- 1/2 Medium Head Cauliflower (Cut Into Small Florets)
- 1 teaspoon of Sea Salt
- 1/2 teaspoon of Freshly Ground Black Pepper
- 1 pound of Sweet Italian Sausage (Ground)
- 1 Medium Carrot (Peeled & Diced)
- 1 Medium Yellow Onion (Chopped)
- 1 tablespoon of Butter
- 2 cloves of Crushed Garlic
- 1 teaspoon of Dried Oregano
- 2 tablespoons of Red Wine Vinegar
- 1 teaspoon of Dried Rubbed Sage
- 1 teaspoon of Dried Basil

Directions:

1. Heat your large-sized saucepan or Dutch oven over a medium-high heat.
2. Add your ground sausage, breaking up your meat.
3. Cook, stirring occasionally until browned and cooked through, Should take approximately 5 minutes.
4. Using your slotted spoon, remove your cooked sausage and allow to drain on a plate covered with your paper towels.
5. Discard the drippings, but do not wash your pan.
6. Melt your butter over a medium heat. When the bubbling subsides, add your onion and carrot.
7. Cook until your onion begins to brown on the edges and becomes somewhat translucent.
8. Stir your garlic into your onion and carrot mixture.

9. Cook for approximately 1 minute.
10. Add your red wine vinegar and cook until syrupy, scraping up any browned bits.
11. Should take about 1 minute.
12. Stir in your oregano, basil, sage and red pepper flakes.
13. Pour in your stock and heavy cream. Increase the heat to a medium high.
14. When your soup reaches a simmer, add your cauliflower and turn the heat down to a medium-low.
15. Simmer uncovered until your cauliflower is fork-tender.
16. Should take about 10 minutes. Stir in your kale and cooked sausage.
17. Cook 1 to 2 minutes longer, or until your kale wilts and your sausage is reheated.
18. Season with your salt and pepper. The amount of salt needed may vary due to variation in brands of broth.Serve!

CPSIA information can be obtained
at www.ICGtesting.com
Printed in the USA
BVHW040901020721
611051BV00016B/437